Dementia Care

Techniques To Improve
The Quality Of Their Life

By

Natalie Johnson

Disclaimer

Please note that I am not a healthcare professional or in any way giving you medical advice. All of the information contained in this book is merely opinionated. You should seek the advice of a healthcare professional before attempting any of the care giving techniques listed in this book.

Table Of Contents

Introduction to Dementia Care

Communication Problems...1

Troubled Behavior 6

Dementia Walk and Wandering..9

Incontinence..13

Agitation 15

Repetitive Actions and Speech 18

Paranoia 20

Bathing..26

Bad Nutrition 31

All Other Areas...36

Conclusion 42

Introduction to Dementia Care

Dementia is a health condition that impairs cognitive function and mental wellbeing. It typically affects older people, although it is not considered to be a normal part of the aging process. Statistics show that over 47 million people around the world suffer from some form of dementia. Not only that, there are over 7 million new dementia cases coming to light ever year as well. Dementia is not a disease, but it can lead to a number of serious diseases of the brain. The most common one is

Alzheimer's disease, which brings about symptoms of memory loss, poor judgment, memory lapses, constant disorientation and difficulty speaking. Eventually, the symptoms will get worse and the patient will end up with a lack of oxygen to their brain. Once this happens, they will be a prime candidate for brain trauma and stroke. The worst part is there is no cure for dementia. That is why it has to be taken seriously and treated as early as possible. That way the person suffering from the condition can slow down the progression of the symptoms.

A person suffering from dementia will not be able to take care of themselves. Their cognitive impairment simply won't sustain their ability to feed, cloth, and exercise themselves like normal people. They will need additional assistance from a close friend, family member or other caregiver. But if you are a loved one, it can be very challenging to care for somebody with dementia that you are close to. For one thing, the person won't be the same anymore.

They will often have mood swings and a completely different personality, which often times is hostile.

If you become offensive around these types of behaviors, then you won't be able to effectively take care of the person. That is why it is always best to have an experienced caregiver in the patient's life in order to offer them the most professional treatment possible. But for those of you who cannot afford to give your loved one a caregiver, you will need this book to guide you through the process of caring for your loved one with dementia.

"Dementia Care" goes over all the care techniques that should be implemented in different situations pertaining to dementia. You will learn care techniques for communication problems, bad behavior, dementia walk and wandering, incontinence, agitation, repetitive actions and speech, paranoia, sleeplessness, bathing, bad nutrition and all other conditions related to dementia. Some of the care techniques for certain symptoms will coincide with the care techniques for other symptoms. Make note of all the symptoms that your patient is currently experiencing and then use this book as a guide to help you care for them.

Eventually, the symptoms of dementia will increase or get worse as the patient gets older. They will likely experience all of the symptoms described in this book at some point in their dementia, whether it is in their early stages or later stages. So always keep this book handy because you never know when you might need it again. But read through it first to become familiar with the symptoms.

That way you can easily recognize the warning signs in your patient and then take action immediately. Good luck!

Communication Problems

Most of us are not trained in caring for a person with dementia. However, you don't have to go to medical school to learn how to do so. You simply have to improve your communication skills and provide a positive atmosphere for the dementia patient. Good communication is very important when being a caregiver because the patient will eventually develop trust and obedience from whatever you say to them. Once you have established this, it will be easier to deal with their difficult behavior and mood swings.

A positive mood is the first step to good communication. No matter what the patient says or does, you cannot become hostile and aggressive with them. You must maintain your composure and stay positive at all times. Dementia patients typically pick up on body language and attitude more than verbal communication. If you use good body language and attitude to communicate your thoughts and feelings, this could become much more effective than speaking words.

Also, your facial expressions and physical interactions with them need to be gentle and sweet. Don't ever manhandle the patients or treat them like animals.

They are still human beings that have feelings and will take great offense to someone who forcibly moves them around like an object. So always be gentle and compassionate whenever you interact with them.

When you are ready to speak to the patient, make sure you get rid of all distractions. This means turning off any televisions or radios that are on in their presence. You should also close the curtains because the outside environment could display something that will take their attention away from you. In fact, you will even want to close the door in the room at certain times because any noises or people from the hallway could become a distraction. You want to get their mind totally focused on you and nothing else. That way they can be totally receptive to everything you say without any interference causing them to lose focus.

If your loved one has gotten to the point where they have trouble remembering who you are, then you need to always state your name and your relationship to that person. For example, if I had a father with dementia then I would greet him with something like, "Hello Father. This is Natalie, your daughter." Of course, I would be seated in front of him while making eye contact. It is important to make eye contact because they need both visual and audio cues in order to help them with their memory. If you were to just come into the room from behind them and say "hi," they probably won't recognize your voice. They will need to see you as well.

Also, when you talk to them make sure you speak slowly and use simple words and sentences. Don't use abbreviations or pronouns when you are talking about someone or something. Always state the name of whom or what you are referring to.

You don't have to raise your voice or tone either. After all, they don't have deafness. They only have dementia. So if you speak to them and they don't understand you, speak the same words again and again until they do understand you. Speak softly with a low pitch when you do this.

If you ask the patient a question then make it simple and easy to answer. Don't ask too many questions at once or questions that are complicated. Ask a question like, "Would you like to wear the blue coat or the black coat?" If you can provide visual cues of what you are asking, then have these available to show them while you ask. Do everything you can to make the questions easier for them to answer. Now when the patient responds, you may have to be patient. Don't expect them to reply or talk as fast as you. They may take many seconds to speak each word. Sometimes they will struggle to say certain words all together. In this situation, it is okay to suggest words to them but make sure you don't talk over them. Suggest the words slowly and give them a chance to repeat your suggestion. That way, it will help them relearn the pronunciation all over again.

Now there are going to be situations where the patient will become upset or aggressive, even if you have been totally calm and patient with them. Perhaps they saw something on television that inflicted a negative emotion in them.

They could have also had a bad dream that upset them. What you have to do in these situations is distract them from the subject. Either that, or change their environment all together. For example, if you go into their room and they appear upset, make a suggestion to go for a walk.

Tell them it is a beautiful day outside and the weather is calm. Give them an incentive to get out of the house and away from whatever is bothering them. But remember to show compassion for whatever is upsetting them. You could say something like, "I'm sorry you are feeling so sad. Hey, I have an idea. Let's go for a walk outside. It is a beautiful day." This will give them an incentive to want to get up and get out.

Dementia patients will often feel anxious and confused about most things. When they try to remember something, they may recall an event that never really happened. More often than not, this will be an event that upsets them to think about. The worst thing you can do is tell them they're wrong about their recollection. This will only enhance their anxiety over the memories they are trying to conjure up.

Instead, just use physical and verbal expressions that offer them reassurance and comfort. You could even hold their hands or give them an occasional hug when they are feeling down. This will make them feel like they are not alone and that you are sympathetic to the recollections that are upsetting them, even though you know they are not true recollections.

Another thing you could do in this situation is help them remember the good times of their past that actually did happen. The amazing thing about dementia patients is that they likely won't remember what happened 50 minutes ago, but they may clearly remember what happened to them 50 years ago. So try mentioning a happy time, like their wedding day or the day their children were born.

Overall, your communication has got to be on the positive side. Some relatives and caregivers like to go a step further by being funny. There is nothing wrong with adding humor to the life of a dementia patient.

Troubled Behavior

In the previous chapter, we mentioned that dementia patients often display aggressiveness and anger towards others. However, they can also behave in a way that is unusual or abnormal. For example, you might go into their room one day and find them asleep on the floor for no apparent reason. Normally you might think that picking them up and putting them on the bed is a good idea, but it is not. You don't want to control their behavior because they will likely just try and resist your attempts. Then they will never trust you again for anything else.

Therefore, you want to try and accommodate their behavior instead. So if the patient insists that they want to sleep on the floor, put a mattress down on the floor. By doing this, you are not changing their behavior. You are just making them more comfortable while accommodating their wishes. This will make them see you in a more positive light as well.

Behavioral issues aren't always a direct symptom of dementia. Sometimes the patient may be experiencing pain or bad side effects from the medications they are taking. That is why you should check with the patient's doctor and have them examined in order to find out where these behavioral issues are coming from. You might think it would be easier just to ask the patient if they are in pain or not.

But you have to remember that dementia patients won't often confide in people about what they need or want. Instead they will express themselves by the actions they take. For example, a patient might take all of the clothes out of their closet every day without saying why. You might think they are looking for a particular article of clothing, but in reality they are just doing something to stay productive. This isn't necessarily a bad thing because it keeps them distracted from their thoughts and negative feelings. As long as they are not causing harm to themselves or others, let them perform these actions on their own.

Troubled behavior could be triggered from something that a person might have said or did, even if it was indirectly targeted towards them. If it was another person then have them leave the room immediately. Either that or get the patient away from the person that caused their bad behavior. Now if you are the one that said or did something unknowingly offensive to the patient, then you will have to develop strategies for managing their behavior. It isn't enough to just apologize and say you're sorry.

You should quickly try to distract them by turning on the television or showing them a picture of something that triggers a happy memory. Often times, the patient will immediately forget about the offensive thing you did or said if they have something pleasant in front of them. However, the same strategies won't work all the time on dementia patients.

Since their troubled behavior could occur from a variety of reasons, you have to be adaptive and develop new strategies all the time for managing their troubled behavior.

If you need assistance coming up with these strategies, search for your nearest Area Agency on Aging by going to www.aoa.gov. You could also try the Caregiver Resource Center at www.caregiver.org.

Dementia Walk and Wandering

Dementia Walk is a symptom of dementia where a patient will aimlessly wander around without any particular reason. They may say they are looking for someone or something, but often times what they are looking for doesn't really exist. Perhaps they have a memory of being a parent and caring for their infant child, so their mind warps back to that period in their life where they think their infant child needs them. This is just one of many examples of what could cause Dementia Walk. Sometimes a dementia patient may also have some need that they aren't sure how to fulfill.

It could be they are looking for a bathroom, water or food for themselves, but don't know where it is. As a caregiver, it is important that you recognize these triggers and assist the patient in fulfilling them. That way they don't wander around too far and get themselves hurt by accident. But in case they do get away, you need to provide them with an ID bracelet of some kind that contains their name and your phone number. If the patient refuses to wear the bracelet it, try sewing the ID information into their clothing. You should also have a recent photograph of them at all times, so you can give it to the police in case they go missing.

Preventive action is the best way to avoid patients from developing Dementia Walk, or at least the best way to reduce it from happening.

For starters, you should give the patient an exercise schedule every day. This could be a simple 30 minute walk outside or even on the treadmill if they prefer to stay indoors. The point is they need to physically exert themselves to some extent because it will satisfy their urges to move around and stay active. The hardest part will be preventing them from wanting to do more physical activity than what is scheduled.

For example, if it is nighttime and you are asleep, you won't be awake to watch over the patient and see if they are wandering around in the dark. That is why you need to install locks on the front and back doors that are either high up on it or close to the ground.

Most dementia patients won't look below or above their eye level, so they won't think to look for the locks in these places. That way you can keep them indoors during the night or anytime you are not around to supervise their actions. However, if you don't like the lock idea then an alternative is to paint the porch black or place a black doormat down. The dementia patient may look at the blackness and think it is some kind of impassable hole or pit. This will make them too scared to want to cross over the blackness because they will be afraid of falling in.

Now you might think that putting locks on the doors is like turning the home into a prison. You only have to put locks on all the doors that allow a person to leave the home.

But for the interior doors, you can use a different approach to help limit the patient's wandering. Try hanging a stop sign on the doors that you don't want them to open. You could also try hanging a curtain over the door in order to mask it.

Even though they would physically be able to get through the door, they won't have the mental capacity to recognize it as a suitable exit. Instead, they will likely obey the stop sign or get confused by the curtain if it is there. There are literally dozens of methods that you could use to confuse a patient into staying in the home rather than wandering outside on their own. There are child-safe plastic covers you can purchase for the doorknobs, which force a person to have to grip the sides inward in order to turn the knob. Dementia patients won't be able to figure this out.

All of the techniques for preventing Dementia Walk that have been discussed so far are fairly inexpensive solutions. But if you really want to keep a close eye on the patient then consider installing a home monitoring or security system for that exact purpose. There are monitoring systems now that have their own Wi-Fi internet connection and cloud hosting service provided by the security company. With this wireless connection, you can actually get real time video feeds downloaded onto your Smartphone from the surveillance cameras set up around your home.

That way if you have to travel away from the patient's home for awhile, you can see how they are doing at any time by watching them on your Smartphone for any location with a Wi-Fi connection. Some of these security companies will even provide you with a GPS device that looks like a watch or clip-on for a belt. So what you could do is clip the device onto the patient's belt.

That way if they ever wander off then you can track their location on your Smartphone from the GPS signal of the device.

Incontinence

As dementia progresses in a patient, they will start to develop incontinence. This is when a person cannot control their bowels or bladder function anymore. In other words, they will involuntarily urinate or release solid waste at anytime during the day. This could become quite embarrassing for them if it occurs in a public setting. Usually patients will be aware that they need to use the bathroom, but their dementia will make it difficult for them to find the bathroom. Even in their own home, they could forget where the bathroom is located. This will result in them having an accident and feeling embarrassed about the whole situation. Once this happens, it could lead to other negative emotions like depression and stress. As the caregiver, you need to constantly be understanding and reassure them that it wasn't their fault. Do everything you can to make them feel comfortable and less embarrassed about their incontinence.

There are always steps you can take to minimize accidents due to incontinence. For example, you could set up a daily routine where the patient has to use the bathroom every two hours. Then try to coincide this with a schedule for fluid intake. That way when they go to the bathroom they will have fluid to release from the bladder. However, do not give the patient any caffeinated drinks or anything that causes diuretic effects because this will increase the level of urine production in their body.

These drinks include tea, coffee, beer or soda. Instead, try to stick with cold water or hot water if possible. If you follow this type of schedule and refrain from giving the patient any diuretic drinks, it will greatly minimize their chances of having an accident. But in case they need to go to the bathroom during an unscheduled time, you don't have to force them to wait for their scheduled time. Just put up signs around the house that will easily guide them to the nearest bathroom.

You can even purchase a commode at any medical supply store and leave it next to the patient's bed for them to use anytime. Commodes are basically portable toilets that you can pick up or wheel around. They are the best thing to have for a dementia patient who has a serious incontinence problem because they can simply use the commode to release their urine or waste at any time.

For further protection of incontinence, you can purchase incontinence pads at your local supermarket or pharmacy. If the patient involuntarily urinates too frequently then you could go to an urologist and have them prescribe a special treatment for dealing with it. But make sure you purchase clothes for the patient that are hard to stain and easy to wash. With all of these preventive techniques of incontinence, there are still going to be situations where they will have accidents in their clothes. You must be prepared for all types of accidents like these.

Agitation

Agitation is one of the more frequent symptoms of dementia. Patients will often become verbally or physically aggressive as a result. By now you should already know how to communicate with a patient when they are in such a state. But, on the sidelines you should still be taking measures to prevent patients from becoming more agitated. Sometimes there are external factors that may be contributing to their agitation and aggressiveness. For example, the junk food and caffeinated drinks they are consuming can result in more anxiety and agitation. This has been proven in people who don't even have dementia. So as you can imagine, giving these food products to a dementia patient will make it even worse.

Dementia sufferers like to have a strict routine. Not only that, but they like to have routine visitors as well. This means they are not comfortable if too many people are in their room. They are also not comfortable when too many objects are added to their room because it will make the atmosphere feel cluttered to them. Then they will shout and become pushy with their caregiver. Therefore, keep the clutter to a minimum and the outside noise as quiet as possible. Let the person chose the people they want to talk to and the music they want to listen to. In fact, you should create a structured routine for them. In the previous chapter, you learned how their trips to the bathroom should become scheduled.

Well this schedule also applies to everything else in their lives. Their television watching, social activities, meals and more should all be set on a schedule. This habitual routine will limit the amount of stress and excitement the patient feels. As a result, they will be much easier for the caregiver to deal with.

Agitation is something that everyone feels at one time or another. You can take preventive measures to reduce the chances of a dementia patient from becoming agitated, but you will never be able to completely prevent it. Therefore, you should always keep dangerous objects out of their reach because you never know when one little thing could set them off in a temper tantrum. You also shouldn't force the scheduled routine upon them. If the patient puts up resistance to any scheduled event or task and prefers to be alone, then allow them to do so. Never force them out of their room and make them do something they don't want to do. Not only would this make dementia patients agitated, it would make any person agitated. So try to be supportive of the patient's independence and let them try to take care of themselves. The only time you should interfere is if they are putting themselves in danger or are risking their health in some way.

If the dementia patient is already agitated and your polite communication attempts have not calmed them down, try to distract them in some way. You could try offering them their favorite snack or turn on the television and show them their favorite TV show.

You may even want to lay out a photo album of their family and let them browse through it. The happy memories and feelings of these distractions will make them forget the reason they were agitated in the first place. As a caregiver, it may take time in the beginning to figure out what objects or methods of distraction will work in these situations. But after awhile, you should be able to make a routine out of these distraction methods.

Repetitive Actions and Speech

One thing you will learn quickly about dementia patients is that their actions and speech are highly repetitive. They will often repeat the same word, question or statement over and over again. This occurs because the dementia patient forgets what they asked or said as little as a few seconds ago. Even though this is completely harmless to the patient themselves, it can become extremely stressful and annoying to the caregiver. If you let this repetitiveness get to your head then it will make you angry and aggressive around the patient. Then they will become agitated and won't trust you anymore to take care of them. So, you have to learn to remain calm and then figure out the triggers that are causing their repetitive behavior.

Repetitive actions and speech may be directly linked to dementia, but they are often triggered by environmental factors. Things like fear, anxiety and boredom will also play a key role in increasing their repetitiveness. The early warning signs of repetitive behavior will action start with their actions instead of their words. For example, a dementia patient may start pulling on their clothing or repeatedly fold the napkins at the dinner table. Strange behavior like this is a definite warning sign. As these repetitive actions progress, it will eventually be noticeable in their verbal language. There isn't much you can do about their actions except to provide a distraction.

Like in the previous chapter, present the patient with an activity that will stir their mind away from their repetitive actions.

When you want to stop repetitive speech, it can be a little more difficult. But what you should never do is remind the patient that they are repeating themselves. This will cause them to get hostile and aggressive. Instead, just let the patient keep repeating themselves and ignore the behavior.

Try to get yourself preoccupied in an activity of your own. As the patient keeps saying the same things, they will notice you are not even paying attention to them because you are caught up in your own activity. This will eventually make them curious enough to want to figure out what the activity is. Then they will likely want to join in on the activity. This could be a board game, television show, crossword puzzle or anything else you can think of.

Overall, a dementia patient never completely gets cured of their repetitive actions and speech. All you can do as a caregiver is place distractions in the way which could make the patient stop talking. Otherwise, you will have to learn to become more tolerant towards this type of behavior. If you cannot handle it then you should find someone else to be their caregiver.

Paranoia

Paranoia is a common occurrence with dementia patients. They will often become highly suspicious of everyone around them, including their loved ones. This will sprout unjustly accusations towards these people. The majority of these accusations have to do with people allegedly trying to kill them or steal from them. No matter how absurd these accusations may sound to a caregiver, to the patient it is very real. If you try to argue or disagree with them, it will just make them more angry and aggressive.

Like mentioned before, never become argumentative with the patient. In fact, it is better not to respond to their accusations at all. If there are other people in the room and they are confused by the accusations, take them aside someplace private and explain to them about the paranoia symptoms of their dementia. That way there are no misunderstandings from others who might make the mistake of taking the patient's accusations seriously.

Dementia patients often think money or personal objects are missing from their possession. The first thing you can do is help them look for the object, and then gradually distract them with a new activity. This will make them forget about what they lost and so they will stop looking for it.

If they don't want to stop looking, then try to figure out where their favorite hiding places are. Dementia patients tend to place objects in certain places and then forget where they put them. This is how things get lost in the first place.

So what you have to do is learn where these common spots are and then check them when they have something go missing. If they have money missing then you could get the patient into the habit of keeping small amounts of money in their handbag or pocket. That way it will be virtually impossible for them to lose the money.

Nonverbal reassurances should work best with a patient experiencing paranoia. Don't be afraid to hug or gently touch their shoulder anytime they are upset over it. When you have to verbally respond to their accusations, always remember to be supportive. Tell the patient that you understand their frustrations over the situation and that you won't let it happen again. If they are worried about their safety then reassure them that you will protect them from harm's way.

Sometimes patients just need someone to hold and comfort them because the paranoia makes them feel lonely and isolated from everyone else in the world. This means you have to be more than just a caregiver. You have to be their friend and family as well if you aren't already.

Sleeplessness

Every person experiences sleeplessness at one time or another. Perhaps you are worried about something and cannot get it out of your mind. This will prevent you from getting any kind of sleep whatsoever. For people who suffer from dementia, sleeplessness could actually occur on a daily basis. Dementia patients are much more prone to anxiety and paranoia, which causes them to think about a lot of things all the time. Some health experts also believe that patients commonly confuse daytime and nighttime. In order to prevent this problem, you need to have clocks all over the patient's home.

They won't typically think of daylight or darkness from the outside as indicating factors. They will just go by what time they feel it is. But if you have clocks on the walls and a watch on their wrist, then it will serve as a constant reminder to them about what time of day it is.

Sleeplessness could occur from a lack of physical activity. We don't just see this in dementia patients, but with normal people as well. Of course, the sleeplessness is a lot more intense with dementia patients. That is why physical activity is crucial to add to their daily routine. You should always try to discourage napping and constant inactivity during the day. If the patient says they want to watch television, suggest exercise or walking outside as an alternative.

The more physical activity they perform during the day, the more exhausted they will feel at nighttime when they are supposed to go to sleep. At this point, their body and mind will be too exhausted to dwell on worries and thoughts. Their only thought will be that they are tired and want to go to sleep. And of course, watch what they eat during the day as well. Avoid giving them sugary or caffeinated foods that will keep them awake, such as candy, coffee, tea, donuts and so on. If they absolutely insist on having these foods, give it to them early on in the day when they just wake up.

By the time it is night, they will be experiencing their caffeine crash and will be too tired to do anything else. But if you give them the food at night, they will be up throughout the night and then crash in the morning. You don't want them to get into this habit, so give them the junk food in the morning or not at all. Preferably, don't give it to them at all.

A caregiver should always make the transition from day to night obvious in the household of the patient. This means opening up the curtains in the morning when the sun comes out and closing the curtains at night when the sun goes down. At nighttime, you will want to use minimal lighting inside the house. Put a nightlight in the patient's room, but nothing too bright or extravagant.

If the interior is too bright then they might mistaken the brightness as sunlight from the outside. So keeping a dimly lit interior setting will avoid this confusion.

It will also deter them from wandering around at night and coming across a dangerous object, like a knife in the kitchen. But just in case they do this, keep locks on the kitchen door and on all areas of the house that contain harmful objects. If you have stairs in the home then always keep the patient on the bottom floor or else they could easily fall down the stairs. Then keep a gate on the bottom of the stairs, so they won't feel compelled to walk up the stairs and risk having an accidental fall.

If all the above methods fail you for some reason or you want additional advice, go seek out a medical professional and ask them what you should do. More often than not, the doctor will prescribe medication to the patient that will help them relax and get a good night's sleep. However, any tranquilizers or sleeping pills you give to a dementia patient could cause them to have more confusion when they wake up the next day.

Ask the doctor to help weigh the pros and cons of giving sleeping pills to a dementia patient. As for you, make sure you get enough sleep as well. You are the caregiver and will need your energy throughout the day in order to handle the patient. If you don't have energy and start napping, then the patient will be left all alone to fend for themselves.

This could cause a whole array of problems for both of you. So always make sure you are getting sleep. If you have to, hire additional help or take shifts with another friend or family member who wouldn't mind being an extra caregiver to the patient.

Bathing

As you spend a lot of time around dementia patients, you will notice that hygiene is not so important to them anymore. It's not that they don't care about their hygiene. They simply forget to take daily actions in order to improve it, such as brushing their teeth, bathing, and changing their clothes. This means the caregiver is going to have to assist the patient in performing these actions for good hygiene. However, this can cause distress for both the caregiver and the patient. Nobody likes to have another person wash them and change their clothes, especially adults. As for the caregiver, it is rather awkward for them to perform these actions on somebody else, especially if it is on a friend or loved one.

Therefore, the caregiver has to work extra hard to make it a comfortable experience for themselves and the patient. On the other hand, if you are just somebody hired to care for a dementia patient who you personally don't know, then bathing and changing them probably won't be too big an issue. But for those who personally do know the patient, you have to resist letting out your true emotions about the situation. Try to keep your cool and don't visually express how uncomfortable the experience is making you feel. If you do then they will resent you quickly and never want you to help them again.

Now if you feel this is something you cannot do, then hire a third party caregiver or certified nursing assistant to take care of these duties.

Most CNA agencies will send a CNA to the caregivers home just to perform a few hours of work, like bathing and changing the patient. Then you can take over after they are done and perform the rest of the normal duties on your own.

If you still prefer to do the bathing on your own, then here are some tips you should follow when working with the dementia patient. First, think about the hygiene routine they used to follow before they got dementia. Did they prefer showers or baths? Did they clean in the morning, at night or both? If it is a female patient, did they like to go to the salon to get their hair washed? What you want to do is recreate their old routine so that it can become somewhat familiar to them. Chances are they will still have memories of doing these things.

They just need a reminder, which is why you will be recreating the hygiene routine in the present. Some dementia patients will even want to bathe on their own, which is fine. All you have to do is make sure they actually start the bathing process and that all the necessary hygiene products are available at their disposal. This means having all the soap bars, shampoo bottles and towels easily accessible around the bathtub. Then when they go to bathe themselves, keep the door open and watch what they are doing.

You should never leave a dementia patient alone in the bathroom because all kinds of accidents could happen where the fall and hurt themselves. So after they are done, smell their hair. If it smells like shampoo then you'll know they actually bathed correctly.

If their hair doesn't smell fresh then suggest that they bathe again. Either that or offer to wash their hair for them. Do everything you can to make the experience as easy and pleasant as possible. This even means putting their bathrobe on them when they come out of the bath or shower.

Caregivers should always prepare the shower or bath for their patient. The reason is because older patients like these tend to be extra sensitive to cold and hot temperatures. You don't want to risk the patient burning themselves or becoming too stunned from icy cold water temperatures. Therefore, set the water to a lukewarm temperature and provide adequate lighting in the bathroom. You will also want to add non-slip bathmats, shower seats and grab bars in the tub. For patients that like to shower but need assistance, have a handheld shower extension available.

This will make it easier for you to wash any part of their body without having to maneuver them around too much. At the same time, they can hold onto the grab bars and secure themselves in place. That way they won't have to move around while washing their body and risk having an accident.

As for washing their hair, try to make this a separate activity from all the other washing. Some patients might respond negatively to being sprayed in the face with a showerhead. So instead, use a cup or a large pitcher and pour lukewarm water over their head. This method of hair washing will be easier for them to endure than being sprayed. Of course, the more expensive alternative is taking them to a salon to get this done.

Patients who are experiencing the later stages of dementia will have a rougher time moving around, let alone get into a bathtub. The whole bathing experience will simply be too traumatic for them to endure. Therefore, you will have to perform something called a "bed bath" on them. Bed baths are when you clean a patient while they are still lying in bed. These are normally performed on patients who are catatonic or comatose because they are bedridden and cannot move around to bathe themselves. With some dementia patients, they won't be able to move around themselves either. So you will need to lightly scrub them down with soap and then rinse off the soap with lukewarm water. Then gently pat them down with a towel to try them off.

You might want to have a nurse show you how to do this because it requires a certain degree of skill, especially when it comes to changing the bed sheets under these conditions.

You will find some dementia patients who can move around on their own, but still hate getting into bathtubs. For these patients, you can perform a towel bath on them as an alternative. This is similar to the bed bath, but in this case you will be using wetted washcloths, towels, and no-rinse soap while they are standing or sitting. You will just gently massage the washcloths and no-rinse soap over the patient's body. Then you will use the towel to dry them off afterwards. If they start to get cold during the process, give them a blanket to wrap around their body so they can stay warm and comfortable. Again, consult a nurse about towel baths if you would like more information on them.

Bad Nutrition

We have already touched upon nutrition somewhat in the previous chapters. You already know that sugary junk foods and caffeinated beverages are very bad to give to a dementia patient. After all, caffeine will increase a person's sleeplessness as well as their anxiety. These are two things you don't want to see happen in a dementia patient who already experiences these symptoms on their own. As for sugary foods, they can also make the patient hyper and easily lose control. Not only that, but they are simply bad for their health anyways.

What you want to focus on is good nutrition for the patient, which is something everybody should be concerned about. The difference between dementia patients and everybody else is dementia patients don't have a choice. Either that or they forget the right foods to consume versus the bad ones. Regular healthy people, on the other hand, do have a choice and are aware of what good foods are. They just fail to make those right choices out of ignorance and low willpower. But you cannot have these attributes when taking care of a dementia patient. You have to put their nutrition on a pedestal and make sure they are eating all natural foods with nothing processed whatsoever. Otherwise, the consequences incurred from poor nutrition could be substantial.

The patient could experience sleeplessness, bladder and bowel problems, irritability, excessive weight loss or weight gain, heart disease and the list just goes on.

A caregiver to a dementia patient has to double as a nutritionist. This means making a schedule for every meal and snack that the patient consumes throughout the day. Not only are you writing down when they consume the food, but you are describing what the food actually is. For example, the breakfast could be Shredded Wheat in Almond Milk with a glass of freshly squeezed orange juice. Something that is natural and healthy will do just fine. Keep this kind of routine up for the rest of the meals and snacks. Also try to stride away from the traditional three meals per day routine because it is actually worse for the body.

Instead, make it five to six small meals per day because this will help their body digest food faster and more efficiently. Meal time should be a special time for the patient. You don't have to just serve them food on a plate and then walk away. Try to liven up the atmosphere with soft music and flower decorations around the room. If there are any loud televisions or radios turned on, turn them off. Meals should be relaxing and stress free for the patient.

Now the next bit of advice has some controversy, but it is logically sound. There is often a debate whether or not you should serve patients finger food or regular seasoned food that requires utensils.

You have to understand that patients won't often have the mental capacity to cut their own food and eat it with a fork. In this situation, you could either cut it up for them or give them finger food. The problem with cutting up the food is it takes away the patient's feeling of independence. They need to be able to feel like they are eating on their own without help. Therefore, do not be afraid to serve them fruit pieces and sandwiches instead of cut up chicken or pasta. Proper table manners do not really matter at this point in their lives. They just need to be able to eat on their own, so do whatever you can to oblige them on that. Of course, when it comes to their beverage you can put a straw in the cup for them to suck up the liquid. They won't have any reservations over that.

As you know by now, dementia patients are constantly feeling lonely and isolated. Meal time is the perfect opportunity to sit down and give them company. You don't necessarily have to eat anything yourself, although it would certainly enhance the mood at the table. Patients may even try to mimic the way you eat and copy every action that you perform. This could be beneficial to you as a caregiver if you need to get your patient to eat their food.

Often times eating with them will overcome their stubbornness to eat because they will want to do what you are doing. However, this doesn't mean you should prepare your favorite foods.

Remember this is all about caring for the patient so you will want to cook their favorite foods.

If they have the ability to tell you what they would like to eat, then you should happily make it for them. Otherwise, ask the patient's family and friends what their favorite food used to be before dementia set in on them. Then you can surprise the patient with a meal that they never expected to have again. But first, make sure they are able to eat the foods. If the patient has dentures or trouble chewing solid foods, then don't grill up a steak with baked potato just yet.

Find out what kinds of foods they are allowed to eat from their family or doctor. Their preference should always come before the preference of the patient because it is for their own good. If you end up serving food and you notice the patient has trouble chewing it, gently move the patient's chin in a gradual chewing motion. Then lightly stroke the outside of their throat to help them swallow it. After that, switch the food to something softer right away.

Believe it or not, dementia patients often experience weight loss problems. If you notice your patient experiencing this then it is okay to serve them high calorie snacks in between their healthy meals. However, this doesn't mean that you give them high calorie meals. You should only give them high calorie snacks because it is just enough calories to sustain their health without it becoming to excessive.

On the other hand, if your patient experiences weight gain then cut out all the high calorie foods and just stick to all natural foods, like fruits, vegetables and white meats. A certified nutritionist can give you further advice if you want more ideas on what to serve your patient.

All Other Areas

There are many problematic symptoms occurring in dementia patients. For this chapter, I have compiled all of the other smaller issues and the best ways to care for them. One issue in particular is a patient who has difficulty dressing on their own. Do not purchase tight clothing for the patient because it will be too difficult for them to put on. Try to purchase looser clothing that has easy-to-use zippers and snappers. Avoid clothing that contains buttons or clothing that requires straps or belts.

The idea is to make the clothing as comfortable as possible for the patient. This means you should remove any clothing from their closet that will be a challenge for them to wear. At this point, they won't have any use for the clothing ever again. So just donate the clothing to Goodwill or some other charitable organization. Then go out and restock their closet with comfortable clothing that they would like to wear. Just pay attention to the kind of loose clothes they already had in the closet and then buy more clothes that are similar to them.

Later on when the patient is ready to get dressed, lay out each article of clothing on their bed in the order they are going to be worn. So first, lay out the underwear. Next lay out the pants, then the shirt and finally the socks. If there are any soiled clothes in the room then remove it immediately and go wash them.

Also, if the patient wants to wear the same clothes again, don't argue with them. Eventually, they will get tired of wearing the same clothes again.

Hallucinations and delusions can occur in dementia patients. These are similar to symptoms of paranoia, but they are a little different. Paranoia is when someone's thought process is influenced by their own fear or anxiety. Hallucinations are simply when people hear or see things that aren't really there. They could be feeling okay one minute, and then the next minute they could be hearing a voice that nobody else hears. As for delusions, these are an underlying result of paranoia. It is when you constantly have false beliefs about other people for no particular reason. All you can do as a caregiver is distract them from their delusions and hallucinations. Don't try to convince them that they are wrong because it will just make them angry. If the severity of their delusions and hallucinations are constant, you will need to get them prescription medication from a doctor. Medication can help enhance the areas of their brain related to memory and judgment. But, this will only be a treatment and not a cure.

Sexual behavior may be noticeable in some dementia patients. You may notice them undressing themselves in public or masturbating out in the open. They may even make lewd remarks or make unreasonable sexual demands.

This sexual behavior can often turn aggressive and violent, especially if the caregiver is a female and the patient is a male. Remember though that this is only happening because of their illness. If the patient had a clean history with no abuse before their dementia, then it is unlikely that their sexual aggression is coming from their own personality. But still, you don't want to take any chances where sexual violence could occur.

That is why you should talk to a doctor the minute you notice this type of behavior in your patient. In the meantime, develop an action plan of what you will do or say in the event that this sexual behavior happens again. Make sure the plan outlines what you will do in each location the patient goes to, such as home, doctor's office, the park or anywhere else in public they might go.

You need a plan or else it could become awkward real fast if you are not prepared. If you can, try to figure out the triggers of this behavior as well. Obviously, you don't want to expose the patient to pornography or any other kind of sexual material. But look and see if other people or certain pictures are triggering this behavior. Sometimes it could be something so insignificant that you might not notice unless you look for it. Once you find the trigger, do what you can do avoid the patient from coming in contact with it again.

An interesting symptom of dementia that often doesn't get talked about is shadowing.

This is when the patient will imitate the actions of their caregiver or simply follow them around wherever they go. The patient may even talk over the caregiver and interrupt every word they try to say. You might think that such actions would be done on purpose, but they are not with dementia suffers. It could be that the patient is just bored or confused about what they should be doing. So as their caregiver, you should comfort them with physical and verbal reassurance. You could also try giving them a small job to do, like folding their laundry or dusting the shelves. Any distraction you can give them will help treat their boredom. It will also make them feel useful and wanted, which will increase their self esteem and self confidence.

Verbal outbursts will be a common occurrence. We have already touched upon this a little in the agitation chapter, but you have to realize that outbursts could happen spontaneously as well. These outbursts could be arguing, cursing, or any kind of threatening manner toward another individual. Remember to stay calm at all times in these situations. Reassure the patient that everything is okay and that they need to remain calm. It is okay to validate whatever feelings they have which are causing the outburst. But what you want to do is try to steer their mind in a different direction by causing a distraction. We have already talked a lot about distractions in this book, but they really are effective for getting the patient's mind to think about something else quickly.

All it could take is a television show or photo album and they will immediately stop their verbal outbursts as quickly as they started them.

Now on a side note, here are some additional tips you should remember when caring for a dementia patient. Firstly, never let them drive a car at all. This should be self explanatory, but some caregivers tend to give in to their patient's demands to drive a car. Even though caregivers are taught to let patients have their independence, this doesn't mean you let them risk endangering themselves or the lives of others. So when it comes to situations like these where they are demanding to do something potentially dangerous, you have to politely tell them that it cannot be done. This doesn't mean you aggressively hold them back and tell them no. Instead, make a valid reason for why they can't do something like drive. Tell them their driver's license was suspended and they can no longer drive a car legally. Something like this might give them a little resistance to drive without you having to be forceful with them.

Finally, you should understand that you as a caregiver are not alone. You are not a medical professional or qualified physician, so don't think that you have to run the whole show. In fact, you will frequently be taking your patient to the doctor to receive their regularly scheduled checkups. When you schedule these checkups, try to make it during a time of day that is less crowded in the doctor's office.

Patients often get nervous around a lot of people they are not familiar with. Plus, when you tell the patient about the appointment you should do so the very same day they have to go. If you tell the patient a week or day before the appointment, they will likely forget about it anyways. Try to prepare a couple of hours in advance. This will be the amount of time you need to feed, bathe, and clothe the patient before the appointment. On your way there, bring along some fun activities and snacks to preoccupy the patient while they wait.

These will also serve as a distraction from the environment around them. That way they will less likely have an outburst that could be embarrassing to both of you. It may even be a good idea to bring a friend along on the trip because you can both share duties. One of you could talk with the doctor and the other could stay with the patient. Of course, the patient will eventually end up having their own private session with the doctor, but you will also want to have your own private session in order to discuss care giving tips with them.

Conclusion

You have made it all the way to the end of the book. By now, you should have plenty of ideas on how to care for dementia patients who are displaying the symptoms outlined in this book. These symptoms include communication problems, bad behavior, dementia walk and wandering, incontinence, agitation, repetitive actions and speech, paranoia, sleeplessness, bathing, bad nutrition and all other conditions. There are a few overall tips that will help you out in most situations.

Remember to always be nice and respectful to the patient. Never try to force anything on them or else they will resent you for it. Try to be a friend to them, whether you personally know them or not. Dementia patients can easily feel alone and isolated from the rest of the world. They may even be aware of their disorder and feel depressed about not being able to function the same way they used to. It is your job as the caregiver to make them feel loved. More importantly, you need to reassure them that getting dementia was not their fault.

Now that you have read the book, I would appreciate it if you left me some feedback on your experiences reading it. Be sure to mention what you have learned about caring for dementia patients and how the information will help you in your life. Perhaps you bought this book for advice on how to care for a loved one with dementia.

Either that or you bought the book because you want to become a professional caregiver and need tips on caring for dementia patients. Now you know the gist of what to do. But as always, consult with a medical professional or healthcare expert before you actually perform these techniques on a real patient. I only provided this information based on scientific research and techniques that I have seen illustrated by other caregivers. The information is meant to give you an idea of what to expect, so be prepared before you take on the duties of a caregiver.

This job isn't necessarily for everyone. If you are attempting to care for your loved one, then you may have an incentive to stick with it out of your love for them. But if you are looking to get a job as a caregiver, then you need to have the right mindset. Not everybody can handle all of the negative behaviors that are often exhibited from a dementia patient. So keep reading this book and let it help you make that choice for yourself.

Thank you and good luck with your future care giving endeavors!

Published by MCJ Publishing
Website: www.book-o-rama.com

You might also be interested in. Available on amazon in Kindle and paperback formats:

Dementia Activities
Keeping Occupied And Stimulated Can Improve The Quality Of Their Life!

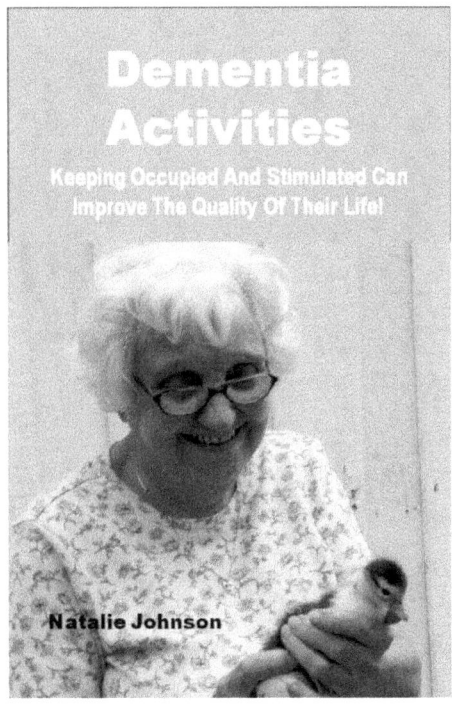